Understanding Osteoporosis

A Comprehensive Guide to Bone Health

Symptoms, Risk Factors, and Strategies for Prevention and Management to Maintain Strong Bones

Graham Julian Oliver

Disclaimer

The information provided in this book, *Understanding Osteoporosis: A Comprehensive Guide to Bone Health: Symptoms, Risk Factors, and Strategies for Prevention and Management to Maintain Strong Bones*, is for informational purposes only. It is intended to enhance your knowledge and understanding of osteoporosis and related topics. This book does not substitute for professional medical advice, diagnosis, or treatment. Always seek the advice of your physician or other qualified health provider with any questions you may have regarding a medical condition or treatment.

The author and publisher of this book make no representations or warranties regarding the completeness or accuracy of the information contained herein. They shall not be liable for any damages arising from the use of this book or reliance on any information contained herein.

The mention of any specific individual, product, website, organization, or other names within this book does not constitute or imply any endorsement or recommendation by the author. All references made are for informational purposes only and do not imply any association or affiliation.

By reading this book, you acknowledge that you understand the nature of the content and agree to take full responsibility for any actions taken based on the information provided.

Table of Contents

About This Book

"Understanding Osteoporosis – A Comprehensive Guide to Bone Health" serves as a crucial resource for anyone seeking to enhance their knowledge of osteoporosis and its implications on overall health. The book begins with a thorough exploration of osteoporosis, defining the condition and illustrating its significant impact on bone health. It highlights the physiological processes that lead to weakened and fragile bones, emphasizing the importance of early diagnosis and ongoing management. With alarming statistics on the prevalence of osteoporosis, the text reinforces the necessity of maintaining strong bones, not only for physical mobility but also for holistic health.

In discussing the importance of bone health, the book delves into the vital roles bones play in the body, supporting structure and facilitating movement. It underscores the intricate connection between bone health and various other health conditions, illustrating how lifestyle choices directly affect bone density. Readers will learn about the lifelong benefits of maintaining robust bone health, and the text offers an overview of preventive measures that can be adopted to enhance bone strength throughout life.

The book further elaborates on the complexities of bone structure and function, examining anatomy, types of bones, and the processes of bone remodeling. It explains how bones adapt to stress and strain and underscores the essential roles of calcium and vitamin D in supporting bone health. The narrative explores the differences between cortical and trabecular bone, the impact of aging, and the effects of hormonal changes on bone metabolism. This foundational knowledge equips readers to better understand the mechanisms of osteoporosis and its progression.

Symptoms and diagnosis of osteoporosis are addressed comprehensively, outlining common signs such as fractures and the importance of routine screening for early detection. The guide discusses various diagnostic tests, including DEXA scans, and the criteria healthcare professionals use to assess bone health. Additionally, it examines risk factors contributing to osteoporosis, ranging from genetic predispositions to lifestyle choices, thereby helping readers identify personal risk factors and understand how to mitigate them.

Nutrition is a critical focus of the guide, detailing the essential dietary components for bone health. It emphasizes the importance of calcium, vitamin D, and other nutrients in maintaining bone strength, while also providing strategies for meal planning to ensure a balanced and bone-healthy diet. Readers will gain insights into the significance of hydration, the effects of excessive sodium, and the roles of vitamins K and C in bone health.

Moreover, the book outlines the importance of physical activity, emphasizing weight-bearing exercises and their benefits for bone density. It offers practical advice for creating effective exercise routines, ensuring safety, and the importance of consulting healthcare providers before embarking on new physical activities. Through a focus on consistency and adapting exercises as needed, the guide empowers readers to incorporate movement into their daily lives to support bone health.

The guide also provides an in-depth overview of medications and treatment options available for osteoporosis management. It discusses the various classes of medications, including bisphosphonates and hormone replacement therapy, as well as the significance of individualized treatment plans. Importantly, it highlights the necessity of regular monitoring and open communication with healthcare providers to manage osteoporosis effectively.

Preventive strategies are a key aspect of the guide, stressing the importance of early intervention and lifestyle modifications to reduce the risk of osteoporosis. The text encourages readers to foster healthy habits, advocate for themselves in healthcare settings, and engage with community resources and support networks to enhance their bone health journey. It addresses common concerns and FAQs, debunking myths and providing clarity on issues surrounding osteoporosis, including exercise safety and dietary choices.

For those living with osteoporosis, the guide offers practical strategies for managing daily life, ensuring safety, and maintaining emotional well-being. It emphasizes the importance of support networks and effective communication with healthcare providers. By empowering readers with knowledge, "Understanding Osteoporosis" serves as a vital tool for individuals seeking to take control of their bone health and navigate the complexities of osteoporosis.

Introduction

Definition of Osteoporosis and Its Impact on Bone Health

Osteoporosis is a medical condition characterized by decreased bone density, making bones fragile and more susceptible to fractures. It occurs when the body loses too much bone mass, doesn't make enough bone, or both. This condition can lead to severe complications, including fractures, especially in the hip, spine, and wrist, which can significantly impair mobility and quality of life.

Understanding osteoporosis is crucial because it often develops silently over many years without noticeable symptoms until a fracture occurs. The impact on bone health is profound, as weakened bones can lead to chronic pain, decreased physical activity, and a higher risk of disability. Therefore, recognizing this condition and its consequences is vital for prevention and management.

Explanation of How Bones Become Weak and Fragile

Bones are living tissues that continuously undergo a process of remodeling, involving the breakdown of old bone and the formation of new bone. In osteoporosis, this balance is disrupted, resulting in a net loss of bone density. Factors contributing to this imbalance include hormonal changes (especially during menopause), inadequate intake of calcium and vitamin D, a sedentary lifestyle, and certain medical conditions or medications that affect bone health.

To combat this weakening process, it's essential to engage in weight-bearing exercises, consume a diet rich in calcium and vitamin D, and avoid smoking and excessive alcohol consumption. By understanding how bones become weak, individuals can take proactive steps to strengthen their skeletal structure and prevent osteoporosis.

Importance of Early Diagnosis and Management

Early diagnosis of osteoporosis is crucial for effective management and prevention of fractures. Health care providers typically utilize bone density tests, such as dual-energy X-ray absorptiometry (DEXA), to assess bone health and determine the risk of fractures. Identifying individuals at risk allows for timely interventions, such as lifestyle modifications or medications, which can help maintain bone density.

Management strategies may include calcium and vitamin D supplementation, weight-bearing exercises, and medications like bisphosphonates. By recognizing the importance of early diagnosis, individuals can take charge of their bone health, significantly reducing their risk of severe complications associated with osteoporosis.

Overview of the Statistics Related to Osteoporosis Prevalence

Osteoporosis is a prevalent condition affecting millions of people worldwide, particularly older adults. According to the World Health Organization, approximately 200 million women globally suffer from osteoporosis, with one in three women and one in five men over the age of 50 experiencing a fracture due to the disease. These statistics highlight the need for increased awareness and proactive measures to address this widespread health issue.

Moreover, it is estimated that by 2025, the number of individuals with osteoporosis will rise significantly due to aging populations. Understanding these statistics emphasizes the importance of preventative strategies and early interventions to mitigate the impact of osteoporosis on public health.

Significance of Maintaining Strong Bones for Overall Health

Maintaining strong bones is essential not only for preventing fractures but also for overall health and well-being. Healthy bones provide support for the body, protect vital organs, and facilitate movement. They also play a crucial role in calcium storage, which is vital for various bodily functions, including muscle contraction and nerve signaling.

To support bone health, individuals should prioritize a balanced diet rich in calcium and vitamin D, engage in regular weight-bearing exercises, and avoid harmful behaviors such as smoking and excessive alcohol consumption. By focusing on maintaining strong bones, individuals can enhance their quality of life and reduce the risk of osteoporosis and related complications.

Why Bone Health Matters?

Role of Bones in the Body's Structure and Movement

Bones serve as the framework of the body, providing structure and support. They protect vital organs, such as the heart and brain, and give shape to our bodies. Bones also work in tandem with muscles and joints to facilitate movement. When muscles contract, they pull on bones, allowing us to perform a wide range of activities, from walking to jumping.

Additionally, bones play a crucial role in the production of blood cells. The bone marrow, found within certain bones, produces red blood cells, white blood cells, and platelets, essential components of our circulatory and immune systems. Strong, healthy bones ensure that our musculoskeletal system operates efficiently, allowing us to maintain mobility and physical independence.

Connection between Bone Health and Other Health Conditions

Bone health is interconnected with various health conditions, influencing overall well-being. Conditions such as osteoporosis lead to weakened bones, increasing the risk of fractures and falls, especially in older adults. Poor bone health can also exacerbate chronic diseases like arthritis, as weakened bones contribute to joint instability and pain.

Moreover, hormonal imbalances, particularly in postmenopausal women, can significantly impact bone density. Low estrogen levels accelerate bone loss, making it crucial to monitor hormone levels and address any imbalances to maintain optimal bone health. Understanding these connections highlights the importance of maintaining strong bones as a foundation for overall health.

How Lifestyle Choices Affect Bone Density

Lifestyle choices significantly impact bone density and overall bone health. Engaging in weight-bearing exercises, such as walking, running, and resistance training, stimulates bone formation and helps maintain bone mass. Regular physical activity increases bone density and strength, making it essential to incorporate exercise into daily routines.

Nutrition also plays a vital role in bone health. Consuming a balanced diet rich in calcium and vitamin D supports bone density. Foods like dairy products, leafy greens, and fatty fish provide essential nutrients for bone formation. Limiting caffeine and alcohol intake is equally important, as excessive consumption can lead to decreased bone density over time.

The Lifelong Benefits of Strong Bones

Maintaining strong bones provides lifelong benefits, starting from childhood through adulthood. Healthy bones support proper growth and development during childhood, laying the groundwork for a strong skeletal system. As we age, strong bones reduce the risk of fractures, which can lead to complications and decreased mobility.

Additionally, strong bones contribute to overall quality of life by promoting physical activity and independence. Maintaining bone health can prevent conditions like osteoporosis and arthritis, ensuring that individuals remain active and capable of engaging in their daily activities without significant limitations.

Overview of Preventive Measures for Maintaining Bone Health

Preventing bone health issues involves adopting a proactive approach to lifestyle and nutrition. Regular physical activity is key; aim for at least 30 minutes of weight-bearing exercise most days. This includes activities such as walking, dancing, and strength training to help build and maintain bone density.

Nutrition plays a vital role as well. Ensure a diet rich in calcium and vitamin D, incorporating foods like yogurt, cheese, nuts, leafy greens, and fortified cereals. Additionally, consider regular check-ups to monitor bone health and discuss potential supplements with a healthcare provider. Making these preventive measures a part of daily life will contribute to long-term bone health.

CHAPTER 1:

Understanding Bone Structure and Function

Explanation of Bone Anatomy and Types of Bones

Bones are complex structures made up of various types of tissue, primarily composed of collagen and calcium phosphate. There are two main types of bone: cortical (or compact) bone, which is dense and forms the outer layer of bones, and trabecular (or spongy) bone, which has a porous structure and is found mainly at the ends of long bones and in the interior of others. Understanding these types is crucial for recognizing how bones function and respond to different stressors.

The anatomy of bones includes several components: the diaphysis (shaft), epiphyses (ends), and the metaphysis (the region between the diaphysis and epiphysis). Each bone is surrounded by a layer called the periosteum, which contains nerves and blood vessels. Knowledge of bone anatomy is essential for maintaining bone health and understanding how fractures or diseases like osteoporosis can affect these structures.

Role of Bones in Supporting the Body and Protecting Organs

Bones provide the framework for the body, supporting weight and facilitating movement. They connect with muscles through tendons and are crucial for maintaining posture and stability. This support allows us to perform everyday activities, from walking to lifting, by providing a structure that withstands physical stress.

In addition to structural support, bones protect vital organs from injury. For example, the skull encases the brain, while the rib cage shields the heart and lungs. Understanding these protective roles emphasizes the importance of maintaining bone health, as weakened bones can lead to increased risk of injury and compromised organ function.

Overview of Bone Remodeling and the Balance of Formation and Resorption

Bone remodeling is a continuous process where old bone tissue is replaced by new bone tissue, involving the activities of osteoblasts (bone formation) and osteoclasts (bone resorption). This balance ensures that bones remain strong and capable of adapting to stress. When remodeling is disrupted, it can lead to conditions such as osteoporosis, where bone density decreases.

To support effective remodeling, regular weight-bearing exercises, a balanced diet, and adequate calcium and vitamin D intake are essential. By engaging in physical activity and providing the body with the necessary nutrients, individuals can promote optimal bone health and maintain a healthy balance between bone formation and resorption.

Importance of Calcium and Vitamin D in Bone Health

Calcium is a crucial mineral for maintaining bone density and strength. It provides the structural component of bone, and inadequate calcium intake can lead to weakened bones and increased risk of fractures. Dairy products, leafy greens, and fortified foods are excellent sources of calcium that should be included in a balanced diet.

Vitamin D plays a vital role in calcium absorption in the body. Without sufficient vitamin D, bones can become brittle and fragile. Sunlight exposure is a natural source of vitamin D, while supplements and foods like fatty fish and fortified cereals can help maintain adequate levels. Prioritizing both calcium and vitamin D is essential for promoting long-term bone health.

How Bones Adapt to Stress and Strain

Bones are dynamic structures that respond to the physical stress and strain placed upon them through a process called mechanotransduction. When bones experience increased loading, such as from exercise, they undergo changes to strengthen and adapt. This adaptation occurs through the remodeling process, where the density and structure of the bone adjust to better withstand future forces.

To encourage this adaptive response, engaging in regular weight-bearing and resistance exercises is crucial. Activities like walking, running, or lifting weights stimulate bone growth and help maintain density, thereby reducing the risk of osteoporosis and fractures. Consistency in physical activity is key to promoting strong, healthy bones.

Differences Between Cortical and Trabecular Bone

Cortical bone, the dense outer layer, provides strength and protection, while trabecular bone, found within the interior, has a more porous structure that supports metabolic activities and aids in nutrient storage. The distinct characteristics of these two types of bone influence how they respond to stress and how susceptible they are to conditions like osteoporosis.

Cortical bone accounts for about 80% of bone mass and is critical for overall strength, whereas trabecular bone, while less dense, is more responsive to changes in diet and physical activity. Understanding these differences can guide individuals in focusing their efforts on maintaining both types through targeted exercise and nutrition strategies.

Impact of Aging on Bone Density

As individuals age, bone density naturally declines due to a decrease in bone formation and an increase in bone resorption. This process is accelerated in postmenopausal women due to a significant drop in estrogen levels, leading to a higher risk of osteoporosis and fractures. Recognizing this age-related decline is essential for proactive health measures.

To mitigate the impact of aging on bone density, adopting a healthy lifestyle is crucial. This includes engaging in regular physical activity, ensuring adequate calcium and vitamin D intake, and avoiding smoking and excessive alcohol consumption. By focusing on these strategies, individuals can preserve bone health and reduce the risk of age-related complications.

Hormonal Influences on Bone Metabolism

Hormones play a significant role in regulating bone metabolism, particularly estrogen, testosterone, and parathyroid hormone. Estrogen helps maintain bone density by inhibiting osteoclast activity, while testosterone is important for bone strength in men. Parathyroid hormone regulates calcium levels and influences bone remodeling.

To support healthy hormonal balance, individuals should prioritize a balanced diet, regular exercise, and stress management. Additionally, consulting with a healthcare provider about hormonal health can help address any potential deficiencies or imbalances that may affect bone health and overall well-being.

Importance of Blood Supply and Nerve Connections to Bones

Bones require a rich blood supply to receive essential nutrients and remove waste products. The blood vessels within the bone tissue, particularly in the periosteum, ensure proper functioning and maintenance of bone health. Adequate blood flow also supports the remodeling process by providing the necessary elements for repair and growth.

Nerve connections to bones are also vital, as they help detect changes in mechanical stress and send signals to initiate remodeling. Maintaining cardiovascular health through regular exercise and a balanced diet is essential to support blood flow to bones, while ensuring the nervous system functions optimally promotes overall bone health and responsiveness to injury.

Effects of Mechanical Loading on Bone Strength

Mechanical loading, or the application of force to bones through physical activity, plays a critical role in enhancing bone strength and density. Weight-bearing exercises stimulate bone formation and can lead to positive adaptations in bone structure. This principle is foundational for preventing bone loss, especially in individuals at risk for osteoporosis.

To maximize the benefits of mechanical loading, individuals should engage in a variety of weight-bearing activities, such as running, jumping, or resistance training. Incorporating these exercises into a regular fitness routine helps promote bone health and resilience, ultimately leading to stronger bones and a reduced risk of fractures.

Relationship Between Bones and Muscles

Bones and muscles work together to enable movement and maintain stability in the body. Muscles attach to bones via tendons, and when muscles contract, they pull on the bones to create motion. This relationship is crucial for overall mobility, as well as for maintaining proper alignment and posture.

To strengthen this relationship, individuals should focus on exercises that build both muscle and bone strength. Resistance training, which challenges muscles and promotes bone density, is particularly effective. By fostering a strong connection between bones and muscles, individuals can enhance overall physical function and reduce the risk of injury.

Role of Bone Marrow in Producing Blood Cells

Bone marrow, located within the cavities of bones, is essential for producing blood cells, including red blood cells, white blood cells, and platelets. This vital function supports the body's ability to transport oxygen, fight infections, and facilitate clotting. Understanding the role of bone marrow emphasizes the interconnectedness of bone health with overall bodily functions.

Maintaining healthy bone marrow requires a nutritious diet rich in vitamins and minerals, such as iron, folic acid, and vitamin B12. Regular physical activity also supports circulation, which is crucial for healthy bone marrow function. By prioritizing these factors, individuals can enhance their bone marrow health and, consequently, their overall well-being.

Overview of Skeletal System Functions Beyond Support

Beyond providing structural support, the skeletal system performs several other essential functions, including facilitating movement, protecting internal organs, storing minerals, and producing blood cells. The bones act as a reservoir for minerals like calcium and phosphorus, which are crucial for various bodily functions, including nerve signaling and muscle contraction.

Additionally, the skeletal system plays a role in the endocrine system by releasing hormones that help regulate mineral balance and bone metabolism. Understanding these diverse functions highlights the importance of maintaining skeletal health through proper nutrition, regular exercise, and lifestyle choices that promote overall wellness.

CHAPTER 2:

Symptoms and Diagnosis of Osteoporosis

Common Symptoms of Osteoporosis, Including Fractures

Osteoporosis often presents with subtle symptoms until a fracture occurs. Common signs include a decrease in height, a stooped posture, and persistent back pain due to vertebral fractures. People may not realize they have osteoporosis until they suffer a fracture from a minor fall or injury, commonly in the hip, wrist, or spine, which can lead to significant pain and disability.

To recognize potential osteoporosis, individuals should be aware of these symptoms and consult a healthcare provider if they experience any sudden or unexplained bone pain. Maintaining a healthy lifestyle with a balanced diet rich in calcium and vitamin D can help support bone strength, but awareness of these symptoms is crucial for early intervention.

Importance of Screening for Early Detection

Screening for osteoporosis is essential for early detection, allowing for timely intervention to prevent fractures. Healthcare professionals recommend that women over 65 and men over 70 undergo regular bone density screenings, especially if they have risk factors such as a family history of the disease or long-term steroid use.

Screening can lead to early diagnosis, enabling individuals to adopt preventive measures or initiate treatment before significant bone loss occurs. Understanding one's bone health status through screening empowers individuals to take proactive steps in maintaining strong bones.

Overview of Diagnostic Tests (DEXA Scans, etc.)

A Dual-Energy X-ray Absorptiometry (DEXA) scan is the most common and reliable test for diagnosing osteoporosis. This non-invasive procedure measures bone mineral density (BMD) at the hip and spine, providing a precise assessment of bone health. The test typically takes about 10-15 minutes and involves lying down on a table while the scanner passes over your body.

Additionally, other tests such as quantitative computed tomography (QCT) may also be used, particularly for those who cannot undergo DEXA scans. It's important to discuss with a healthcare provider which test is appropriate based on individual health needs and circumstances.

Signs of Bone Loss to Watch For

Individuals should monitor for signs that may indicate bone loss, such as increased susceptibility to fractures, a noticeable change in posture, or a loss of height over time. These signs can be subtle but serve as vital indicators that it's time to seek medical advice regarding bone health.

Regular self-assessments, such as maintaining awareness of one's balance and strength, can help catch potential issues early. If any unusual changes are observed, consulting a healthcare professional for further evaluation is essential for effective management.

Risk Assessment Tools for Osteoporosis

Several risk assessment tools are available to help determine an individual's likelihood of developing osteoporosis. The FRAX tool, for example, calculates the 10-year probability of a major osteoporotic fracture based on clinical risk factors and bone density measurements.

Using these tools, healthcare providers can identify individuals at higher risk and recommend appropriate preventive strategies. Understanding one's risk factors can also motivate lifestyle changes that support bone health, such as diet, exercise, and avoiding smoking and excessive alcohol consumption.

Differences between Osteoporosis and Osteopenia

Osteoporosis and osteopenia are related but distinct conditions. Osteopenia is characterized by lower-than-normal bone density but does not yet meet the criteria for osteoporosis. Individuals with osteopenia are at an increased risk of developing osteoporosis if no preventive measures are taken.

Recognizing the difference is crucial for intervention. If diagnosed with osteopenia, individuals should focus on lifestyle modifications, including weight-bearing exercises and adequate calcium and vitamin D intake, to strengthen their bones and potentially halt further decline.

Understanding the Role of Medical History in Diagnosis

A comprehensive medical history is crucial for diagnosing osteoporosis. Healthcare providers will inquire about personal and family medical histories, including any previous fractures, hormonal changes, medication use (such as corticosteroids), and lifestyle factors like diet and physical activity.

This information helps identify risk factors that contribute to bone health. By understanding one's medical background, healthcare professionals can provide personalized recommendations for prevention and management, making it essential for individuals to discuss their health history openly during consultations.

Importance of Physical Examinations in Assessing Bone Health

Physical examinations play a vital role in assessing bone health and identifying signs of osteoporosis. During an examination, healthcare providers may check for height loss, spinal deformities, and balance issues that could indicate weakened bones.

Regular physical examinations allow healthcare professionals to track changes over time and recommend appropriate interventions. Individuals should maintain regular check-ups to ensure their bone health is monitored and managed effectively.

Diagnostic Criteria Used by Healthcare Professionals

Healthcare professionals use specific diagnostic criteria to identify osteoporosis. The World Health Organization (WHO) defines osteoporosis based on a T-score from a DEXA scan, with a T-score of -2.5 or lower indicating osteoporosis.

Understanding these criteria helps individuals comprehend their bone health status. If diagnosed with osteoporosis, patients can then work with their healthcare provider to create a management plan that includes lifestyle changes and potential treatments.

Interpretation of Bone Density Test Results

Interpreting bone density test results involves understanding the T-score and Z-score. The T-score compares an individual's bone density to that of a healthy young adult, while the Z-score compares it to someone of the same age and sex. A T-score of -2.5 or lower indicates osteoporosis, while osteopenia is indicated by a score between -1 and -2.5.

Patients should discuss their test results with their healthcare provider to understand the implications fully. Knowing one's scores can inform necessary lifestyle adjustments and treatment options to maintain or improve bone health.

Importance of Family History in Risk Assessment

Family history is a significant factor in assessing osteoporosis risk. Individuals with a family history of osteoporosis or fractures are more likely to develop the condition themselves, making it essential to discuss family health backgrounds with healthcare providers.

Understanding one's genetic predisposition can guide proactive measures for prevention. If osteoporosis runs in the family, individuals should focus on lifestyle changes, such as diet and exercise, to help mitigate their risk.

Role of Biomarkers in Diagnosing Osteoporosis

Biomarkers are substances in the body that can indicate bone turnover and health status. Blood and urine tests can measure levels of specific biomarkers, such as osteocalcin and bone-specific alkaline phosphatase, to assess bone formation and resorption.

Monitoring these biomarkers can help healthcare professionals track the effectiveness of treatments and the overall health of bones. Individuals may benefit from these tests as part of a comprehensive approach to managing osteoporosis.

Next Steps after Diagnosis: Treatment Options

After a diagnosis of osteoporosis, individuals should discuss treatment options with their healthcare provider. Common treatments include bisphosphonates, hormone therapy, and calcium and vitamin D supplementation, aimed at reducing fracture risk and improving bone density.

Creating a personalized treatment plan is vital. This plan may include lifestyle modifications, such as dietary changes and exercise programs, along with medications, to ensure a comprehensive approach to managing bone health.

CHAPTER 3:

Risk Factors for Osteoporosis

Overview of Genetic Predisposition to Osteoporosis

Genetic predisposition plays a crucial role in osteoporosis risk. Individuals with a family history of osteoporosis or fractures are more likely to develop the condition themselves. Genes influence bone density and quality, as well as how our bodies respond to various environmental factors, such as diet and physical activity. If osteoporosis runs in your family, it's important to be proactive about monitoring bone health.

To address genetic risks, regular bone density screenings are essential. Those with a family history should discuss their risk factors with a healthcare provider and consider lifestyle modifications early on. Maintaining a balanced diet rich in calcium and vitamin D, along with regular weight-bearing exercises, can help mitigate some genetic risks

Importance of Age and Gender as Risk Factors

Age and gender significantly affect osteoporosis risk. As we age, bone density naturally decreases, particularly after the age of 30. Women are especially vulnerable post-menopause due to a sharp decline in estrogen an level, which protects bone density. Understanding these factors can empower individuals to take preventive measures earlier in life.

To counteract these risks, individuals should focus on preventive strategies starting in their 20s and 30s. This includes engaging in regular strength-training exercises and ensuring adequate calcium and vitamin D intake throughout life. Regular check-ups can also help monitor bone density and overall health.

Impact of Hormonal Changes (e.g., Menopause)

Hormonal changes, especially during menopause, can drastically increase the risk of osteoporosis in women.

The decline in estrogen leads to increased bone resorption, outpacing the formation of new bone. This imbalance can result in significant bone loss, making it vital for women to understand this risk factor as they approach menopause.

Managing this risk involves consulting with healthcare providers about possible treatments, such as hormone replacement therapy (HRT). Lifestyle modifications, including a bone-healthy diet and regular exercise, are also crucial. Women should prioritize maintaining bone strength during and after the transition into menopause.

Role of Lifestyle Factors: Diet, Exercise, and Smoking

Lifestyle choices have a profound impact on bone health. A balanced diet rich in calcium and vitamin D, alongside regular physical activity, promotes strong bones. Conversely, smoking has been linked to decreased bone density and increased fracture risk, making it essential to avoid or quit smoking for better bone health.

To cultivate healthy habits, individuals should aim for a balanced diet and incorporate weight-bearing exercises like walking, jogging, or resistance training into their routine. It's also beneficial to avoid smoking and seek support to quit if necessary, thereby enhancing bone health and overall well-being.

Influence of Medications on Bone Health

Certain medications can adversely affect bone health, increasing the risk of osteoporosis. Corticosteroids, for example, can decrease bone formation and increase resorption, leading to a greater risk of fractures. It's essential to be aware of how prescribed medications may impact your bone density.

If you are taking medications known to affect bone health, consult your healthcare provider about alternatives or additional preventive measures. This may include taking supplements to counteract bone loss or regular bone density testing to monitor changes.

Open communication with your doctor is key to managing your bone health effectively.

Connection between Chronic Diseases and Osteoporosis Risk

Chronic diseases, such as rheumatoid arthritis, diabetes, and hyperthyroidism, can significantly increase the risk of developing osteoporosis. These conditions can interfere with the body's ability to maintain healthy bone density or may involve medications that contribute to bone loss.

To manage this risk, it is crucial for individuals with chronic diseases to have regular check-ups with their healthcare provider. This includes monitoring bone density and discussing specific lifestyle adjustments or treatments that can help protect bone health. Staying informed about your health status can lead to better bone care.

Nutritional Deficiencies: Calcium and Vitamin D

Calcium and vitamin D are critical nutrients for bone health. Calcium strengthens bones, while vitamin D aids in calcium absorption. Deficiencies in these nutrients can lead to decreased bone density and an increased risk of fractures, making it vital to ensure adequate intake.

To incorporate these nutrients into your diet, focus on consuming dairy products, leafy greens, and fortified foods for calcium, and fatty fish or fortified cereals for vitamin D. If dietary sources are insufficient, consider speaking with a healthcare provider about supplementation to maintain optimal levels for bone health.

Importance of Weight Management for Bone Health

Maintaining a healthy weight is essential for bone health. Underweight individuals are at a higher risk for osteoporosis due to reduced bone mass, while being overweight can increase stress on the bones and lead to fractures. Striking a balance is vital for maintaining strong bones.

To achieve and maintain a healthy weight, individuals should focus on a balanced diet combined with regular physical activity. Engaging in strength training can also enhance bone density while promoting overall body strength. Setting realistic weight goals and consulting with a nutritionist may further support bone health.

How Excessive Alcohol Consumption Affects Bones

Excessive alcohol consumption negatively impacts bone health, increasing the risk of osteoporosis. Alcohol can interfere with the body's calcium balance and hormonal levels, leading to decreased bone formation and increased resorption. Limiting alcohol intake is crucial for maintaining healthy bones.

To protect your bones, aim to limit alcohol consumption to moderate levels. For those who drink, this generally means up to one drink per day for women and two for men. Creating a support system or seeking help if alcohol consumption becomes a challenge can further safeguard bone health.

Effects of Sedentary Lifestyle on Bone Density

A sedentary lifestyle is a significant risk factor for osteoporosis. Lack of physical activity can lead to decreased bone density and strength, as bones need regular stress from exercise to maintain their health. Encouraging movement and exercise is vital to preventing bone loss.

To combat a sedentary lifestyle, individuals should aim to incorporate at least 30 minutes of weight-bearing exercise most days of the week. This can include walking, dancing, or resistance training. Simple adjustments, like taking stairs instead of elevators, can also contribute to better bone health over time.

Overview of Ethnic and Racial Variations in Risk

Ethnic and racial backgrounds can influence osteoporosis risk, with variations in bone density and fracture rates observed across different populations. For instance, Caucasian and Asian individuals are at a higher risk compared to African Americans, who generally have higher bone density. Understanding these differences can help tailor preventive strategies.

Individuals should consult with healthcare providers about their specific risk based on ethnic or racial background. This includes discussing appropriate screening and preventive measures. Being informed about personal risk factors allows for better management and prevention of osteoporosis.

Role of Physical Activity in Reducing Risk

Physical activity is one of the most effective strategies for reducing osteoporosis risk. Regular weight-bearing and resistance exercises help to build and maintain bone density, while also improving balance and coordination to prevent falls. Staying active is essential for strong bones.

To incorporate physical activity into daily life, individuals should aim for a mix of aerobic and strength-training exercises. Activities like walking, jogging, dancing, and lifting weights can be beneficial. Setting specific fitness goals and finding enjoyable activities can encourage consistency and enhance bone health.

Importance of Understanding Personal Risk Factors

Understanding personal risk factors for osteoporosis is crucial for effective prevention and management. Factors such as family history, lifestyle choices, age, and medical conditions can all influence bone health. Being informed allows individuals to take proactive steps to protect their bones.

To assess personal risk, individuals should consider keeping a health journal that includes family history, lifestyle habits, and any existing health conditions. Consulting with healthcare providers for personalized assessments and recommendations can lead to targeted strategies for maintaining strong bones.

CHAPTER 4:

Nutrition for Bone Health

Importance of Calcium and Dietary Sources

Calcium is a vital mineral for maintaining strong bones and preventing osteoporosis. Adults should aim for 1,000 to 1,200 mg of calcium daily, depending on age and gender. To meet this requirement, incorporate dairy products like milk, yogurt, and cheese into your diet. For those who are lactose intolerant or prefer non-dairy options, consider fortified plant-based milks, leafy green vegetables, almonds, and tofu.

To enhance calcium intake, aim to spread your consumption throughout the day. For instance, start your day with a calcium-fortified cereal, enjoy a yogurt-based snack in the afternoon, and include leafy greens in your dinner. Cooking methods like steaming can also help preserve the calcium content in vegetables, ensuring you maximize your intake.

Role of Vitamin D in Calcium Absorption

Vitamin D is crucial for calcium absorption in the intestines and helps maintain adequate serum calcium and phosphate levels for bone health. The recommended daily intake is 600 to 800 IU, which can be achieved through sun exposure, diet, and supplements. Foods rich in vitamin D include fatty fish (like salmon and mackerel), fortified dairy products, and egg yolks.

To ensure you are getting enough vitamin D, aim for about 15 to 30 minutes of sun exposure several times a week, depending on your skin type and local climate. If sunlight is limited, consider fortified foods or supplements, especially in winter months, to maintain optimal levels for bone health.

Overview of a Bone-Healthy Diet

A bone-healthy diet is well-balanced and includes various food groups to ensure sufficient nutrients for bone strength. This diet emphasizes fruits, vegetables, whole grains, lean proteins, and healthy fats, focusing on foods that are high in calcium, vitamin D, and other essential nutrients.

To construct your bone-healthy meal plan, incorporate a rainbow of fruits and vegetables for their antioxidants and nutrients. Opt for whole grains instead of refined grains, and choose lean protein sources like fish, poultry, legumes, and nuts. Avoid overly processed foods that can lead to nutrient deficiencies.

Importance of Protein for Bone Health

Protein plays a significant role in bone health by helping to maintain bone density and strength. Adults should consume around 46 grams for women and 56 grams for men daily. Good sources of protein include lean meats, poultry, fish, eggs, dairy products, legumes, and nuts.

To ensure adequate protein intake, incorporate a source of protein in every meal and snack. For example, add beans to salads, include chicken in stir-fries, and snack on Greek yogurt or nuts. Balancing your protein intake with other nutrients is essential for overall health and bone maintenance.

Foods to Include for Optimal Bone Strength

For optimal bone strength, include foods rich in calcium, vitamin D, magnesium, and phosphorus. Dairy products, leafy greens, nuts, seeds, fatty fish, and fortified foods are excellent choices. These foods not only provide essential nutrients but also support overall health.

To maximize benefits, aim to include a variety of these foods daily. For breakfast, consider oatmeal topped with almonds and yogurt; for lunch, a spinach salad with salmon; and for dinner, a vegetable stir-fry with tofu. This variety ensures a broad spectrum of nutrients necessary for strong bones.

Role of Magnesium, Phosphorus, and Potassium

Magnesium, phosphorus, and potassium are essential minerals that contribute to bone health. Magnesium aids in converting vitamin D into its active form, while phosphorus helps build and maintain bones. Potassium contributes to maintaining bone density by reducing calcium loss from bones.

Include foods high in these minerals in your diet, such as nuts, seeds, legumes, whole grains, and leafy green vegetables. For example, snack on a handful of mixed nuts, add quinoa to salads, or enjoy a side of baked sweet potatoes. These small changes can significantly impact your bone health over time.

Importance of Hydration for Overall Health

Hydration is crucial for overall health, including bone health. Proper hydration supports cellular function and nutrient transportation, which are essential for maintaining bone density and strength. Aim for at least 8 cups of water daily, adjusting based on activity levels and climate.

To stay hydrated, carry a water bottle and set reminders to drink water throughout the day. Incorporate hydrating foods like cucumbers, oranges, and watermelon into your diet. Herbal teas and low-sugar beverages also count toward your daily fluid intake, helping you meet your hydration goals.

Foods to Limit for Better Bone Health

Certain foods can negatively affect bone health and should be limited. High amounts of caffeine, alcohol, and processed foods can lead to calcium loss and weaken bones. Additionally, excessive sugar can contribute to inflammation, further impacting bone density.

To improve your bone health, reduce intake of soda, sugary snacks, and excessive caffeine. Instead, opt for water, herbal teas, and nutrient-dense snacks like fruits, nuts, and yogurt. This shift can enhance your overall diet and promote stronger bones.

Overview of Supplements: When They Are Necessary

While a balanced diet is the best way to obtain essential nutrients, supplements may be necessary for some individuals, especially if dietary sources are insufficient. Common supplements for bone health include calcium, vitamin D, and magnesium, which can help fill nutrient gaps.

Before starting any supplements, consult with a healthcare professional to determine your specific needs and the appropriate dosages. If you're not getting enough nutrients from your diet due to restrictions or health conditions, targeted supplementation can support bone health effectively.

Impact of Excessive Sodium on Bone Health

Excessive sodium intake can lead to calcium loss through urine, increasing the risk of osteoporosis. The recommended daily limit for sodium is around 2,300 mg. High-sodium diets can be found in processed foods, canned goods, and fast food, which can undermine bone health over time.

To reduce sodium intake, focus on fresh, whole foods, and read labels on packaged items for sodium content. Cooking at home allows you to control the amount of salt you use, and using herbs and spices can enhance flavor without relying on sodium.

Role of Vitamins K and C in Bone Health

Vitamins K and C are vital for bone health and play unique roles in maintaining bone density. Vitamin K is essential for bone mineralization and may help prevent fractures, while vitamin C is necessary for collagen production, which is crucial for bone structure.

To ensure adequate intake, include foods rich in these vitamins, such as leafy greens (for vitamin K) and citrus fruits or bell peppers (for vitamin C). Incorporate these foods into your meals—add spinach to smoothies or enjoy orange slices as a snack—to support your bone health.

Importance of a Balanced Diet in Preventing Osteoporosis

A balanced diet is fundamental in preventing osteoporosis by providing all essential nutrients required for bone strength. Focus on a diverse range of foods from all food groups, including fruits, vegetables, whole grains, lean proteins, and healthy fats.

Make meal planning easier by creating a weekly menu that incorporates these foods. For example, plan meals that feature a variety of colorful vegetables, whole grains like brown rice or quinoa, and lean proteins such as chicken or beans to ensure you are meeting your nutritional needs effectively.

Strategies for Meal Planning to Support Bone Health

Effective meal planning can greatly support bone health by ensuring that you consistently consume nutrient-dense foods. Start by creating a weekly menu that includes a variety of calcium-rich foods, fruits, vegetables, and whole grains. This will help you avoid last-minute unhealthy choices.

Use a shopping list based on your meal plan to guide your grocery trips, making it easier to stick to healthy options. Prepare meals in batches and freeze portions for busy days, ensuring you always have nutritious meals ready to go.

CHAPTER 5:

Exercise and Physical Activity

Importance of Weight-Bearing Exercises for Bone Strength

Weight-bearing exercises are essential for building and maintaining bone density. These activities, which include walking, jogging, dancing, and weightlifting, force your bones to work against gravity. This process stimulates bone formation and helps counteract the natural bone loss that occurs with age or osteoporosis. Incorporating these exercises into your routine can significantly improve your bone health and reduce the risk of fractures.

To start, aim for at least 30 minutes of moderate weight-bearing exercise on most days of the week. You can break this down into shorter sessions if needed. It's important to choose activities that you enjoy, making it more likely that you will stick with your routine over time. Always listen to your body, and gradually increase the intensity and duration of your workouts as you build strength.

Overview of Resistance Training and Its Benefits

Resistance training, also known as strength training, involves exercises that cause your muscles to work against an external resistance. This can include weights, resistance bands, or your own body weight. The benefits of resistance training extend beyond muscle strength; it also helps improve bone density, balance, and overall functionality. By strengthening muscles, you can better support your skeletal structure and reduce the risk of falls.

To get started with resistance training, consider using resistance bands or light weights. Focus on major muscle groups, aiming for two to three sessions per week. Perform exercises like squats, lunges, and push-ups, ensuring you maintain proper form to prevent injury. As you progress, you can gradually increase the resistance to continue challenging your muscles.

Types of Exercises Beneficial for Osteoporosis Prevention

Several types of exercises can effectively prevent osteoporosis. High-impact exercises like jumping or running can help stimulate bone growth, while low-impact activities like swimming and cycling improve cardiovascular health without stressing the bones. Additionally, exercises that focus on muscle strength, such as weightlifting, and balance, such as tai chi, are crucial for reducing fall risk and improving overall stability.

Incorporate a mix of these exercises into your weekly routine for optimal results. For example, you could schedule weight training on Mondays and Wednesdays, reserve high-impact activities for Tuesdays and Thursdays, and finish your week with flexibility and balance training on weekends. This variety will help keep your workouts engaging and ensure that you're addressing different aspects of bone health.

Role of Flexibility and Balance Exercises in Fall Prevention

Flexibility and balance exercises play a vital role in preventing falls, which is especially important for individuals with osteoporosis. Improved flexibility can enhance your range of motion and reduce the risk of injuries during daily activities. Balance exercises, such as standing on one leg or practicing yoga, strengthen stabilizing muscles, helping you maintain control and stability.

To integrate flexibility and balance training into your routine, dedicate a few minutes each day to stretching major muscle groups and practicing balance exercises. Consider joining a yoga or tai chi class to learn proper techniques in a supportive environment. Regular practice not only helps prevent falls but also improves overall mobility and quality of life.

Recommendations for Safe Exercise Practices

Safety is paramount when exercising with osteoporosis. Always start slowly and gradually increase the intensity of your workouts to avoid injury. Use proper footwear to provide support and stability during exercises, and ensure your workout space is free from hazards. Avoid high-impact activities and movements that involve twisting or bending at the waist, as these can increase the risk of fractures.

Additionally, warm up before exercising and cool down afterward to prepare your body for physical activity. Listen to your body; if you experience pain or discomfort during an exercise, stop and consult a healthcare professional. Keeping a journal of your exercises can help you track your progress and identify any patterns that may require adjustments.

Importance of Consistency in Physical Activity

Consistency in physical activity is key to maintaining bone health and preventing osteoporosis. Regular exercise not only builds and preserves bone density but also enhances muscle strength, balance, and overall physical fitness. Establishing a routine helps create healthy habits that can last a lifetime, making it easier to incorporate exercise into your daily life.

To stay consistent, choose activities you enjoy and set realistic goals. Consider working out with a friend or joining a class to stay motivated. Creating a weekly exercise schedule can help you prioritize physical activity, ensuring that you allocate specific times for workouts amidst your other responsibilities.

How to Create an Effective Exercise Routine

Creating an effective exercise routine involves setting specific, measurable, attainable, relevant, and time-bound (SMART) goals. Start by assessing your current fitness level and determining what types of exercises you enjoy. Include a variety of activities that target different aspects of fitness, such as weight-bearing exercises, resistance training, flexibility, and balance exercises, to keep your routine well-rounded.

Once you have identified your goals and preferred activities, plan your workouts for the week, allowing for rest days to promote recovery. Keep your routine flexible so you can adapt to changes in your schedule or energy levels. Tracking your workouts can help you stay motivated and accountable as you work towards your goals.

Importance of Consulting with Healthcare Providers Before Starting

Consulting with healthcare providers before starting an exercise program is crucial, especially for individuals with osteoporosis or other health concerns. Your doctor can provide guidance on safe activities, help assess your risk factors, and tailor an exercise program to your specific needs. They may also recommend physical therapy if you need additional support or instruction.

When meeting with your healthcare provider, be prepared to discuss your exercise history, any medications you're taking, and any existing health conditions. This information will help them offer personalized recommendations and ensure that you approach exercise in a way that minimizes risks and maximizes benefits.

Role of Physical Therapy in Managing Osteoporosis

Physical therapy plays a significant role in managing osteoporosis by providing tailored exercise programs designed to strengthen bones and improve overall mobility. A physical therapist can assess your individual needs and create a plan that includes safe exercises to build strength, flexibility, and balance. This professional guidance is especially important for individuals at high risk for fractures.

During physical therapy sessions, you'll learn proper techniques and receive feedback to ensure you perform exercises safely and effectively. Regular visits can help monitor your progress and make adjustments as needed, giving you the confidence to exercise independently while minimizing the risk of injury.

Safety Tips for Exercising with Osteoporosis

When exercising with osteoporosis, safety should always be your top priority. Begin with low-impact activities and avoid exercises that involve sudden or jerky movements, heavy lifting, or twisting motions. Use proper equipment, such as supportive shoes, and consider using mats or padding to cushion your workouts and prevent falls.

It's also wise to have a buddy system in place, particularly during high-risk exercises. Ensure you have someone nearby who can assist you if needed. Remember to hydrate before, during, and after exercise, and pay attention to your body, stopping any activity that causes pain or discomfort.

Benefits of Walking and Other Low-Impact Activities

Walking is one of the simplest and most effective low-impact activities for maintaining bone health. It promotes cardiovascular fitness while being gentle on the joints and bones. Aim for at least 30 minutes of walking most days of the week. You can easily incorporate this into your routine by walking in your neighborhood, using a treadmill, or joining a walking group for added motivation.

In addition to walking, other low-impact activities such as swimming, cycling, and water aerobics can provide excellent cardiovascular benefits without putting excessive strain on your bones. These activities help maintain a healthy weight and enhance muscle tone, contributing to better overall health and reducing the risk of fractures.

Connection Between Physical Activity and Overall Health

Physical activity has a profound impact on overall health, extending beyond bone health. Regular exercise can help manage weight, reduce the risk of chronic diseases, improve mental health, and boost mood. Engaging in physical activities fosters a sense of well-being and can enhance your quality of life as you age.

To reap these benefits, strive to incorporate a variety of exercises into your weekly routine. Balance aerobic activities with strength training and flexibility exercises to promote comprehensive health. This holistic approach to fitness will not only support your bones but also improve your overall physical and mental well-being.

Importance of Adapting Exercises as Needed

Adapting exercises is crucial for maintaining safety and effectiveness, especially for individuals with osteoporosis. As you progress or experience changes in your health, it's important to modify your exercise routine to meet your current abilities. This may involve reducing the intensity of certain exercises, choosing alternative activities, or consulting with a professional for tailored guidance.

Listening to your body and recognizing when to adjust your exercises can help prevent injuries and ensure that you continue to benefit from your routine. Keep an open line of communication with your healthcare providers and physical therapists to discuss any concerns or changes in your condition, allowing for a safe and effective exercise journey.

CHAPTER 6:

Medications and Treatment Options

Overview of Medications Used to Treat Osteoporosis

Osteoporosis medications aim to strengthen bones and reduce fracture risk. The primary categories include bisphosphonates, hormone replacement therapy, and newer agents like monoclonal antibodies. Each type works differently to slow bone loss or enhance bone formation, and they are prescribed based on individual health needs and risk factors.

Before starting any medication, it's crucial to consult a healthcare provider who can explain the various options available and their potential effects. Understanding the purpose and expected outcomes of each medication helps patients make informed decisions about their treatment plans.

How Bisphosphonates Work and Their Benefits

Bisphosphonates are a class of drugs that inhibit the activity of osteoclasts, the cells responsible for bone resorption. By slowing down this process, bisphosphonates help maintain bone density and lower the risk of fractures. Commonly prescribed bisphosphonates include alendronate, risedronate, and zoledronic acid.

To take bisphosphonates effectively, patients should follow specific guidelines: take the medication on an empty stomach with a full glass of water, and remain upright for at least 30 minutes afterward. This helps enhance absorption and reduce gastrointestinal side effects.

Role of Hormone Replacement Therapy in Management

Hormone replacement therapy (HRT) involves supplementing estrogen or progesterone to help protect bone density, particularly in postmenopausal women. Estrogen plays a significant role in maintaining bone health, and its decline during menopause can lead to accelerated bone loss. HRT can significantly reduce fracture risk when used appropriately.

To consider HRT, individuals should discuss their personal and family medical histories with their healthcare providers. Providers will weigh the benefits of bone protection against potential risks, such as an increased chance of blood clots or certain cancers.

Overview of Newer Medications for Osteoporosis

Recent advancements in osteoporosis treatment have led to the development of newer medications like denosumab and romosozumab. Denosumab is a monoclonal antibody that reduces bone resorption by inhibiting RANKL, a protein involved in osteoclast formation. Romosozumab, on the other hand, both increases bone formation and decreases resorption, making it a dual-action therapy.

These newer medications are often reserved for patients who do not respond well to traditional treatments or those at high risk of fractures. Administered via injection, they typically require monitoring and follow-ups to evaluate effectiveness and any side effects.

Importance of Discussing Risks and Benefits with Healthcare Providers

When considering osteoporosis treatment options, it's vital for patients to have open discussions with their healthcare providers regarding the potential risks and benefits of each medication. This dialogue ensures that patients understand how each treatment aligns with their specific health needs and personal circumstances.

Patients should come prepared with questions about side effects, long-term impacts, and alternative treatments. Having this information allows for a collaborative approach to developing an effective osteoporosis management plan tailored to individual preferences and health goals.

Role of Calcium and Vitamin D Supplements in Treatment

Calcium and vitamin D are crucial for maintaining strong bones, as they support bone density and overall skeletal health. Calcium is the primary mineral found in bones, while vitamin D aids in calcium absorption and bone remodeling. For many individuals, dietary sources may not provide sufficient amounts, necessitating supplementation.

To maximize benefits, individuals should aim for a balanced diet rich in dairy products, leafy greens, and fortified foods. When taking supplements, it's important to follow recommended dosages and consult with a healthcare provider to determine individual needs based on dietary intake and bone health status.

Importance of Individualized Treatment Plans

Each individual with osteoporosis has unique health considerations, which is why individualized treatment plans are essential. Factors like age, gender, medical history, and lifestyle all play a role in determining the best approach to managing bone health. A personalized plan increases the likelihood of successful treatment outcomes.

To create an effective treatment plan, patients should work closely with their healthcare providers, sharing all relevant medical information. Regular reviews of the plan can help adjust medications, supplements, and lifestyle changes based on progress and new developments in bone health.

How to Manage Side Effects of Osteoporosis Medications

Many osteoporosis medications can cause side effects, such as gastrointestinal discomfort or flu-like symptoms. To manage these effects, patients should follow the prescribed guidelines for each medication, including taking them with food or at specific times to minimize discomfort.

If side effects persist or become severe, patients should communicate with their healthcare providers. In some cases, switching medications or adjusting dosages may be necessary to improve tolerance and ensure continued treatment effectiveness.

Role of Lifestyle Modifications in Conjunction with Medication

In addition to medications, lifestyle modifications play a vital role in osteoporosis management. Weight-bearing exercises, such as walking or strength training, help improve bone density and strength. A balanced diet rich in nutrients, avoiding smoking, and limiting alcohol intake also contribute to better bone health.

Incorporating these lifestyle changes can enhance the effectiveness of medications and reduce fracture risk. Patients should aim for regular physical activity and make dietary adjustments that support bone health, while also discussing any new exercise programs with their healthcare providers.

Importance of Regular Monitoring and Follow-Ups

Regular monitoring and follow-up appointments are crucial for assessing the effectiveness of osteoporosis treatments. Healthcare providers may conduct bone density tests and review medication adherence and lifestyle changes. These evaluations help determine if adjustments are needed to optimize bone health.

Patients should maintain consistent communication with their healthcare providers and report any new symptoms or concerns. Regular monitoring ensures that treatments are effective and that any potential issues are addressed promptly.

Understanding the Duration of Treatment and Its Importance

The duration of osteoporosis treatment can vary based on individual responses to medication and overall bone health. Some patients may require long-term treatment to maintain bone density, while others might benefit from periodic reassessments to determine if medication can be paused or adjusted.

Understanding the treatment timeline helps patients stay engaged in their bone health management. Regular discussions with healthcare providers about the duration and goals of treatment can clarify expectations and motivate adherence to the prescribed plan.

Alternatives for Those Who Cannot Take Traditional Medications

For individuals who cannot tolerate traditional osteoporosis medications due to side effects or other medical conditions, alternatives exist. Options may include lifestyle changes, dietary adjustments, or specific non-pharmacological interventions that focus on improving bone health naturally.

Consulting with healthcare providers about alternative treatments ensures that patients receive guidance tailored to their unique situations. Exploring options like exercise programs, nutritional counseling, or complementary therapies can help manage osteoporosis effectively without traditional medications.

Role of Comprehensive Care in Managing Osteoporosis

Comprehensive care involves a multidisciplinary approach to osteoporosis management, integrating medical, nutritional, and lifestyle support. Healthcare providers, including physicians, dietitians, and physical therapists, work together to create holistic treatment plans that address all aspects of bone health.

Patients are encouraged to engage actively in their care by participating in discussions about treatment options and following through on lifestyle recommendations. This collaborative approach fosters a supportive environment for managing osteoporosis and enhancing overall well-being.

CHAPTER 7:

Preventing Osteoporosis

Importance of Early Intervention for Bone Health

Early intervention in bone health is crucial to preventing osteoporosis and related fractures. This involves identifying risk factors, such as family history or hormonal changes, and implementing preventive measures. Regular bone density tests, especially for those over 50 or with risk factors, can help detect issues early and guide necessary lifestyle changes.

Taking proactive steps, like incorporating calcium and vitamin D into your diet or starting a weight-bearing exercise routine, can significantly enhance bone density. Engaging with healthcare providers early allows individuals to create a tailored plan that includes nutritional guidance and exercise, laying a strong foundation for long-term bone health.

Lifestyle Changes That Can Reduce Risk

Making lifestyle changes is essential for reducing the risk of osteoporosis. Regular physical activity, particularly weight-bearing exercises like walking, jogging, or strength training, helps strengthen bones. A balanced diet rich in calcium and vitamin D, found in dairy products, leafy greens, and fortified foods, is also vital for bone health.

Additionally, avoiding smoking and limiting alcohol consumption can further mitigate risk. Establishing these healthy habits early in life promotes bone density and reduces the likelihood of developing osteoporosis later on.

Importance of Regular Health Check-Ups

Regular health check-ups play a critical role in maintaining bone health. These appointments allow healthcare providers to monitor bone density, assess risk factors, and make necessary recommendations. For those at risk, screenings can help catch osteoporosis before it progresses, enabling timely intervention.

During these visits, patients should discuss their family history, lifestyle choices, and any symptoms they may experience. Following medical advice, including recommended supplements or medications, can significantly enhance bone health and prevent fractures.

Role of Education in Osteoporosis Prevention

Education is vital in preventing osteoporosis by empowering individuals with knowledge about bone health. Understanding the importance of nutrients like calcium and vitamin D, as well as the impact of lifestyle choices, helps individuals make informed decisions. Resources such as workshops, online courses, and informational pamphlets can provide valuable insights into maintaining strong bones.

Additionally, educating the community about osteoporosis fosters a culture of prevention. This can involve partnering with local health organizations to host seminars, distribute literature, and promote awareness campaigns focused on the importance of bone health.

Strategies for Creating a Bone-Healthy Environment

Creating a bone-healthy environment involves making conscious choices at home and in the community. This includes ensuring access to nutritious foods rich in calcium and vitamin D, as well as promoting physical activity through safe and accessible spaces. Families can create a culture of health by participating in activities like hiking, biking, or attending fitness classes together.

In the workplace, employers can promote a bone-healthy environment by offering wellness programs that include fitness challenges or nutrition workshops. Encouraging colleagues to participate in physical activities during breaks fosters a supportive atmosphere where everyone can prioritize their bone health.

Importance of Community Resources and Support Groups

Community resources and support groups play an essential role in osteoporosis prevention and management. Local organizations often provide educational materials, workshops, and access to healthcare professionals who specialize in bone health. Joining a support group can offer emotional support and practical advice for individuals navigating osteoporosis.

These groups can also facilitate social connections, making it easier for participants to share experiences and challenges. By engaging with community resources, individuals can access vital information and encouragement, making it easier to implement healthy changes in their lives.

Role of Advocacy in Raising Awareness About Osteoporosis

Advocacy is crucial for raising awareness about osteoporosis and promoting bone health initiatives. Individuals can advocate for better access to screenings, educational programs, and supportive resources within their communities. By participating in or organizing awareness campaigns, individuals can help spread the message about the importance of preventing osteoporosis.

Additionally, collaborating with healthcare professionals and local organizations can enhance advocacy efforts. This can include lobbying for policy changes that support bone health initiatives and encouraging public health campaigns that emphasize the importance of osteoporosis prevention.

Importance of Fostering Healthy Habits in Children

Fostering healthy habits in children is essential for lifelong bone health. Encouraging physical activity through sports and outdoor play helps build strong bones from an early age. Parents and caregivers can also model healthy eating by providing meals rich in calcium and vitamin D, making these nutrients a regular part of children's diets.

Moreover, educating children about the importance of bone health can empower them to make informed choices as they grow. Engaging them in discussions about nutrition and exercise fosters a proactive approach to maintaining healthy bones throughout their lives.

How to Address Myths and Misconceptions About Osteoporosis

Addressing myths and misconceptions about osteoporosis is vital for effective prevention and management. Common myths, such as osteoporosis only affecting older women, can lead to a lack of awareness in other demographics. Educating the public through accurate information helps dispel these myths and promotes a broader understanding of osteoporosis risk factors.

Encouraging open conversations about osteoporosis can also help individuals feel more comfortable seeking help and information. By providing clear and factual resources, communities can combat misinformation and foster a more informed public.

Importance of Self-Care in Bone Health

Self-care is essential for maintaining bone health and preventing osteoporosis. This involves prioritizing activities that promote physical and mental well-being, such as regular exercise, a balanced diet, and stress management techniques. Individuals should establish a routine that includes weight-bearing exercises, healthy meals, and time for relaxation to support overall bone health.

Additionally, self-care practices like mindfulness, meditation, and proper sleep hygiene contribute to overall health, which can indirectly benefit bone density. By prioritizing self-care, individuals empower themselves to take charge of their bone health and reduce the risk of osteoporosis.

Overview of Workplace Initiatives for Health Promotion

Workplace initiatives for health promotion can significantly enhance employees' awareness of bone health. Employers can implement wellness programs that focus on nutrition, exercise, and regular health screenings. This may include offering fitness classes, providing healthy snacks, or organizing health fairs that emphasize the importance of osteoporosis prevention.

By fostering a culture of health within the workplace, employers can encourage employees to make positive lifestyle changes. This collective approach not only improves individual health but also enhances overall productivity and morale in the workplace.

Encouraging Family Support for Lifestyle Changes

Encouraging family support is vital for successfully implementing lifestyle changes related to bone health. Families can work together to create a supportive environment that promotes healthy eating and regular physical activity. This can include cooking nutritious meals together, participating in exercise routines, and setting shared health goals.

Additionally, having family members on board can boost motivation and accountability. When everyone is committed to fostering healthy habits, it becomes easier to maintain lifestyle changes that benefit bone health and prevent osteoporosis.

CHAPTER 8:

Living with Osteoporosis

Strategies for Managing Daily Life with Osteoporosis

Managing daily life with osteoporosis involves creating a routine that prioritizes bone health. Incorporate weight-bearing exercises, such as walking or gentle resistance training, into your daily schedule to strengthen bones. It's also vital to maintain a well-balanced diet rich in calcium and vitamin D, as these nutrients support bone density. Consider consulting with a nutritionist to create meal plans that meet your specific dietary needs.

Additionally, stay organized by using tools like calendars or apps to track your exercise and dietary goals. Plan your daily activities to include sufficient rest periods, as fatigue can increase the risk of falls. Utilize resources such as occupational therapy to learn techniques for safe movement and self-care, ensuring that you navigate daily tasks with confidence and reduced risk.

Importance of Safety Measures to Prevent Falls

Implementing safety measures is crucial in preventing falls, which can lead to serious injuries in individuals with osteoporosis. Begin by assessing your home for hazards such as loose rugs, poor lighting, and clutter. Remove or secure these items to create a safer environment. Installing grab bars in bathrooms and using non-slip mats can also enhance safety in high-risk areas.

Moreover, wear supportive footwear that provides stability, and avoid slippery surfaces when walking. Consider using assistive devices like canes or walkers if needed, as these tools can significantly reduce the risk of falls. Regularly reviewing and adjusting safety measures is essential, as your needs may change over time.

How to Adapt Living Spaces for Safety

Adapting living spaces for safety involves making practical changes that promote mobility and independence. Start by decluttering rooms, especially walkways and stairs, to eliminate tripping hazards. Ensure that frequently used items are within easy reach to minimize the need for stretching or climbing. Installing adequate lighting in every room, particularly in hallways and staircases, can also help prevent accidents.

Consider using furniture that is sturdy and at a comfortable height to aid in sitting and standing. If necessary, modify bathrooms with raised toilet seats and walk-in showers to enhance accessibility. These adjustments can create a safer living environment that allows you to maintain independence while reducing the risk of injury.

Overview of Coping Strategies for Emotional Health

Coping with osteoporosis can be emotionally challenging, but implementing effective strategies can enhance your emotional well-being. Begin by practicing mindfulness techniques, such as meditation or deep breathing exercises, which can help reduce anxiety and promote relaxation. Engaging in hobbies and activities you enjoy can provide a positive outlet for stress and improve your overall mood.

Additionally, consider journaling to express your feelings and track your progress in managing osteoporosis. This reflective practice can help you identify triggers for stress and develop healthier coping mechanisms. Seeking professional support through therapy or counseling can also provide valuable tools for managing emotional health during this journey.

Role of Support Networks in Managing Osteoporosis

Establishing a strong support network is vital in managing osteoporosis effectively. Reach out to family members and friends for emotional support, and consider joining support groups where you can connect with others facing similar challenges. Sharing experiences and strategies can empower you and provide a sense of community, reducing feelings of isolation.

Additionally, involve your support network in your health journey by educating them about osteoporosis. By understanding the condition, they can offer practical assistance, such as accompanying you to appointments or participating in safe physical activities together. A well-rounded support system can significantly enhance your motivation and resilience.

Importance of Educating Family and Friends

Educating family and friends about osteoporosis is essential for fostering understanding and support. Share information about the condition, including symptoms, treatment options, and the importance of lifestyle changes. This knowledge can help your loved ones become more empathetic and encourage them to participate actively in your care and well-being.

Furthermore, inform them about specific challenges you may face, such as the risk of falls or the need for dietary adjustments. By involving them in discussions about your health, you can create an environment where they feel comfortable supporting your journey and advocating for your needs in social situations.

How to Communicate with Healthcare Providers Effectively

Effective communication with healthcare providers is crucial for managing osteoporosis successfully. Prepare for appointments by writing down questions and concerns in advance. Be open and honest about your symptoms, lifestyle, and any challenges you face in adhering to treatment plans. This transparency will help your provider tailor recommendations that align with your individual needs.

Additionally, take notes during consultations to ensure you understand the information provided. Don't hesitate to ask for clarification on medical terminology or treatment options. Building a collaborative relationship with your healthcare team can lead to better outcomes and increased confidence in managing your condition.

Importance of Keeping Track of Medications and Appointments

Keeping track of medications and appointments is vital for effective osteoporosis management. Create a medication schedule, using pill organizers or reminder apps, to ensure you take medications consistently. Discuss with your healthcare provider about the best times to take each medication, as some may have specific requirements for optimal absorption.

Equally important is maintaining a calendar for medical appointments and follow-ups. Regular check-ups enable your healthcare team to monitor your bone health and adjust treatment as necessary. Consider involving a family member or friend to help remind you of appointments, ensuring that you remain proactive in your healthcare management.

Ways to Celebrate Milestones in Bone Health Management

Celebrating milestones in bone health management is essential for maintaining motivation and a positive outlook. Recognize significant achievements, such as completing a rehabilitation program, reaching a fitness goal, or maintaining a balanced diet for a specific period. Acknowledging these successes can boost your confidence and reinforce healthy habits.

Consider organizing small celebrations, such as inviting friends for a healthy meal or treating yourself to a favorite activity. Documenting your progress in a journal or through photos can serve as a visual reminder of your journey, helping you stay focused on your goals and fostering a sense of accomplishment.

Importance of Staying Informed About New Research

Staying informed about new research on osteoporosis can enhance your understanding and management of the condition. Subscribe to reputable health publications, follow relevant organizations, or join online forums to receive updates on the latest findings and treatment options. Knowledge empowers you to make informed decisions about your health and adapt your management strategies accordingly.

Moreover, discuss any new information with your healthcare provider to see how it may apply to your situation. Being proactive about your health can lead to improved outcomes and increased confidence in managing osteoporosis effectively.

Role of Stress Management in Overall Health

Managing stress is crucial for overall health, especially for individuals with osteoporosis. Chronic stress can negatively impact bone density and overall well-being. Incorporate stress-relief techniques such as yoga, meditation, or regular physical activity into your daily routine. These practices can help lower cortisol levels, improving mood and promoting relaxation.

Additionally, prioritize self-care by engaging in activities that bring you joy and fulfillment. Whether it's spending time with loved ones, pursuing hobbies, or practicing mindfulness, fostering a balanced lifestyle can enhance your emotional resilience and contribute to better bone health.

Strategies for Maintaining Social Connections

Maintaining social connections is vital for emotional health, particularly for those managing osteoporosis.

Make an effort to schedule regular outings with friends or family, whether it's a coffee date, a walk in the park, or a game night at home. These interactions can provide emotional support and reduce feelings of isolation.

Additionally, consider joining community groups or clubs that align with your interests. Engaging in social activities can help you form new friendships while promoting a sense of belonging. Staying socially active contributes positively to mental well-being and can encourage you to stay motivated in your bone health journey.

Importance of Self-Advocacy in Health Care Decisions

Self-advocacy is a crucial component of effective healthcare management for individuals with osteoporosis. Educate yourself about your condition, treatment options, and potential side effects to make informed decisions. Feel empowered to voice your preferences and concerns during medical appointments, as this can lead to better personalized care.

Moreover, don't hesitate to seek second opinions if you feel uncertain about a proposed treatment plan. Trust your instincts and prioritize your health needs. By actively participating in your healthcare decisions, you can establish a collaborative relationship with your providers, leading to more effective management of osteoporosis.

CHAPTER 9:

Common Concerns and FAQs

Understanding the Myths
Surrounding Osteoporosis

Osteoporosis is often misunderstood, with many believing it only affects older women. In reality, it can impact anyone, regardless of gender or age, leading to misconceptions about who should be concerned. It's crucial to dispel these myths by educating individuals about the importance of bone health throughout life and that risk factors, such as family history and lifestyle choices, apply to everyone.

Additionally, many people mistakenly think that osteoporosis symptoms are immediately noticeable, when in fact, it often develops silently over many years. Understanding that proactive measures can help in maintaining strong bones is vital, including regular screenings and lifestyle modifications that can lower risk.

Clarification of Dietary Misconceptions

Diet plays a pivotal role in bone health, yet many individuals harbor misconceptions about the nutrients needed to maintain strong bones. Calcium and vitamin D are essential, but people often overlook other important nutrients like magnesium, vitamin K, and zinc, which also contribute to bone density. To improve bone health, it is recommended to include a variety of foods in your diet, such as leafy greens, nuts, fish, and dairy products.

To ensure adequate nutrient intake, individuals should consider keeping a food diary to track their daily consumption and identify any gaps. Consulting with a registered dietitian can provide personalized guidance on dietary choices that support bone health, making it easier to implement necessary changes.

Questions about the Safety of Physical Activity

Many individuals with osteoporosis worry that physical activity could lead to fractures or further injury. However, regular, safe exercise is essential for building and maintaining bone density. Weight-bearing and resistance exercises, such as walking, dancing, or lifting weights, can strengthen bones and improve balance, reducing the risk of falls.

To begin a safe exercise routine, consult a healthcare provider or physical therapist who can tailor a program specific to your needs. Start slowly, gradually increasing intensity while focusing on proper form to avoid injury. Incorporating activities like yoga or tai chi can also enhance flexibility and stability.

Importance of Addressing Emotional Health Concerns

The diagnosis of osteoporosis can lead to anxiety and depression for many individuals. Emotional health plays a significant role in overall well-being and can influence one's motivation to engage in preventive measures. Recognizing and addressing these emotional concerns is crucial for successful management of bone health.

To support emotional health, consider joining support groups or engaging in counseling to discuss fears and frustrations. Incorporating stress-reducing practices such as meditation, mindfulness, and regular social interactions can also improve mental health and provide a supportive environment for managing osteoporosis.

Questions about Long-Term Medication Use

Many individuals prescribed medication for osteoporosis have concerns about the long-term effects and safety of these drugs. While some may experience side effects, it's essential to weigh these against the benefits of preventing fractures. Regular follow-ups with healthcare providers can help assess the effectiveness of medication and make necessary adjustments.

For those worried about long-term use, discussing alternative therapies, such as lifestyle changes or supplements, may provide additional options. Staying informed about the latest research on osteoporosis medications can empower individuals to make educated decisions regarding their treatment plans.

Addressing Fears Related to Fractures and Injuries

Fear of fractures can prevent individuals from participating in activities they once enjoyed. Understanding that while osteoporosis increases fracture risk, many preventive strategies can reduce this risk is important. Maintaining a healthy lifestyle, including balanced nutrition and regular exercise, helps build strength and stability.

Education is key; learning proper techniques for lifting and avoiding high-risk activities can significantly decrease the likelihood of injury. Consulting with a physical therapist can provide tailored strategies to navigate daily activities safely, alleviating fears related to fractures.

Common Inquiries about Supplements and Nutrition

Supplements can be a helpful addition to one's diet for improving bone health, yet many individuals are uncertain about which ones to take. Calcium and vitamin D are the most commonly recommended, but other nutrients like omega-3 fatty acids and probiotics can also support bone density. It's crucial to assess dietary intake before relying solely on supplements.

To determine the right supplements, consult with a healthcare provider who can recommend appropriate dosages based on individual needs and dietary gaps. Regularly reviewing and adjusting supplement use ensures optimal bone health without unnecessary excess.

Questions Regarding Screening Frequency

Understanding how often to get screened for osteoporosis is essential for early detection and management. Generally, individuals should begin screenings at age 50 or earlier if they have risk factors such as family history or previous fractures. Regular follow-ups can help monitor bone density and determine the effectiveness of lifestyle changes or treatments.

It is advisable to discuss personalized screening schedules with a healthcare provider, who can evaluate individual risk factors and provide recommendations. Staying proactive about screenings is vital for maintaining bone health and preventing complications associated with osteoporosis.

Addressing Concerns about Aging and Bone Health

Aging is often associated with a decline in bone density, but it is essential to recognize that it doesn't mean inevitable deterioration. Individuals can take proactive steps throughout their lives to maintain strong bones, including engaging in regular exercise, eating a balanced diet, and avoiding smoking and excessive alcohol consumption.

Understanding that it's never too late to improve bone health can motivate individuals to adopt healthier habits. Encouraging lifestyle changes and staying informed about aging-related bone health can empower individuals to take control of their well-being as they age.

Importance of Understanding Individual Health Risks

Everyone's risk for osteoporosis varies based on genetics, lifestyle, and other health factors.

Understanding personal risk factors—such as family history, previous fractures, and hormonal changes—can guide individuals in implementing preventive measures tailored to their unique situation.

To gain insight into personal health risks, consider discussing concerns with a healthcare provider, who can provide personalized assessments and recommendations. Taking a proactive approach by understanding and addressing these risks can significantly improve bone health outcomes.

Common Misconceptions about Osteoporosis Treatments

Many individuals have misconceptions regarding osteoporosis treatments, believing they are only necessary for older adults or that they are ineffective. In reality, treatments can benefit individuals of various ages, especially those at risk. It's essential to dispel these myths through education and discussions with healthcare providers.

Being open to various treatment options, including medications and lifestyle changes, can empower individuals to find the most effective approach for their situation. Regularly reviewing treatment plans ensures that individuals remain informed and engaged in their osteoporosis management.

Questions about the Impact of Genetics on Bone Health

Genetics plays a significant role in bone health, influencing an individual's risk for osteoporosis. While certain genetic factors are beyond control, lifestyle choices can mitigate these risks. Engaging in regular exercise, consuming a balanced diet, and avoiding harmful habits can help strengthen bones regardless of genetic predispositions.

To better understand personal genetic risks, individuals can consider discussing family health histories with their healthcare providers. This information can help tailor preventive strategies that account for genetic factors, promoting proactive bone health management.

Importance of Seeking Professional Advice for Concerns

When in doubt about bone health or osteoporosis, seeking professional advice is crucial. Healthcare providers can offer tailored recommendations based on individual risk factors and health histories, guiding individuals toward appropriate treatments and preventive measures.

Regular check-ups allow for ongoing assessments of bone health, enabling adjustments to lifestyle or treatment plans as needed. Empowering individuals to take charge of their health through professional guidance can significantly improve outcomes and enhance overall well-being.

Common Concerns

Addressing Fear of Fractures and Injury

Many individuals with osteoporosis experience a heightened fear of fractures and injuries, which can significantly impact their daily lives. This fear often stems from the understanding that bones are more fragile, leading to anxiety about engaging in physical activities. To address this, it's crucial to educate oneself about safe movement strategies and consider participating in supervised exercise programs tailored for those with osteoporosis. These programs can help build confidence and strength, reducing the fear of falling and sustaining injuries.

Additionally, incorporating balance and flexibility training into your routine can further minimize the risk of falls. Simple practices like tai chi or yoga can improve coordination and awareness of body positioning, making it easier to navigate daily tasks. Engaging with support groups or speaking to a healthcare professional can also provide reassurance and tips for safely managing daily activities.

Concerns about Medication Side Effects

Concerns about medication side effects are common among individuals managing osteoporosis. Many fear that the benefits of medications may be outweighed by potential adverse effects, such as gastrointestinal issues or other health complications. To alleviate these concerns, it's essential to have open discussions with healthcare providers about the risks and benefits of prescribed medications. They can provide tailored information and alternative options if side effects are a significant concern.

Additionally, maintaining a journal to track any side effects experienced can be beneficial. This record can help both the patient and the healthcare provider make informed decisions about medication adjustments or alternative therapies. Staying informed about new osteoporosis treatments and participating in discussions with healthcare professionals can empower individuals to manage their condition effectively.

Questions Regarding the Effectiveness of Supplements

Questions regarding the effectiveness of dietary supplements for bone health often arise, especially concerning calcium and vitamin D. While supplements can play a role in supporting bone health, they should not replace a balanced diet. To ensure maximum effectiveness, focus on obtaining nutrients from whole foods such as dairy products, leafy greens, and fortified foods, and use supplements as an adjunct when necessary. Consulting a healthcare provider before starting any supplement regimen is crucial for determining the appropriate dosage and form.

Moreover, regular monitoring of nutrient levels through blood tests can help assess if supplementation is needed. Combining a nutritious diet with adequate sunlight exposure can enhance vitamin D levels, further supporting calcium absorption. Engaging in physical activity can also stimulate bone strength, making it essential to view supplements as part of a holistic approach to bone health.

Fear of Losing Independence Due to Bone Health Issues

The fear of losing independence due to osteoporosis is a significant concern for many individuals. This fear can lead to a reluctance to engage in activities or seek help, which can inadvertently worsen bone health. To combat this, it is vital to develop a supportive network of family, friends, and healthcare providers who can assist in maintaining independence while ensuring safety. Encouragingly, many programs focus on adaptive techniques that allow individuals to remain active and involved in their communities.

Creating an individualized exercise plan that emphasizes strength, balance, and mobility can significantly bolster confidence and autonomy. Occupational therapy may also provide strategies to modify the home environment, making it safer and more accessible. By taking proactive steps to manage bone health, individuals can maintain a sense of independence and control over their lives.

Understanding the Balance Between Activity and Safety

Understanding the balance between staying active and ensuring safety is critical for individuals with osteoporosis. While regular physical activity is essential for maintaining bone density, it is crucial to choose low-impact, weight-bearing exercises that minimize the risk of injury. Activities like walking, swimming, and cycling can be excellent choices that promote cardiovascular health without excessive strain on the bones. Consulting a healthcare provider or physical therapist can help design a personalized exercise plan that incorporates safe activities tailored to individual capabilities.

Moreover, incorporating flexibility and balance exercises into daily routines can enhance stability and reduce fall risk. Simple adjustments, such as using supportive footwear, modifying the home environment, and avoiding high-risk activities, can further enhance safety. Understanding one's limits and gradually increasing activity levels while paying attention to body signals will promote a healthier and safer lifestyle.

FAQs

What Are the Early Signs of Osteoporosis?

Early signs of osteoporosis may be subtle and can include symptoms such as bone pain, fractures that occur more easily than expected, and noticeable changes in posture, like stooping or a hunched back. To stay vigilant, individuals should pay attention to any sudden or unexplained pains, especially in the back or hips, and should seek medical advice if these symptoms occur. Regular check-ups and communication with healthcare professionals can facilitate early detection and intervention.

Being proactive about bone health by maintaining a balanced diet, engaging in weight-bearing exercises, and avoiding smoking and excessive alcohol consumption can also help minimize the risk of developing osteoporosis. Recognizing these early signs allows individuals to take preventive measures and seek appropriate treatment before the condition progresses.

Can Osteoporosis Be Cured?

Osteoporosis is a chronic condition that cannot be cured; however, it can be effectively managed and prevented through various lifestyle changes and medications. Emphasizing nutrition, particularly calcium and vitamin D intake, regular exercise, and maintaining a healthy lifestyle are essential strategies for managing osteoporosis. Consulting with healthcare providers for personalized management plans can empower individuals to take control of their bone health.

Engaging in bone-strengthening exercises and adopting dietary changes can significantly improve bone density and overall health. While osteoporosis management requires ongoing attention and care, many individuals successfully lead active lives with the right strategies in place.

What Foods Are Best for Bone Health?

Foods that promote bone health are primarily rich in calcium, vitamin D, and protein. Dairy products like milk, cheese, and yogurt are excellent sources of calcium, while leafy greens (such as kale and broccoli) and fish (like salmon and sardines) provide essential nutrients for bone maintenance. To incorporate these foods, consider adding leafy green salads to meals, snacking on yogurt, and including fish in weekly menus.

Moreover, fortified foods such as orange juice and cereals can also boost vitamin D levels. Maintaining a well-rounded diet rich in these nutrients is vital for supporting bone strength and overall health. Regularly consulting with a nutritionist can further refine dietary choices to meet individual bone health needs.

How Often Should I Get Tested for Osteoporosis?

The frequency of osteoporosis testing varies based on individual risk factors, including age, family history, and existing health conditions. Generally, women over 65 and men over 70 should undergo screening, while younger individuals with risk factors may require earlier testing. To establish a personalized screening schedule, it's essential to have discussions with healthcare providers, who can provide recommendations tailored to your specific health profile.

Staying informed about your bone health is crucial, and regular screening can help track changes in bone density over time. If osteoporosis is diagnosed, healthcare providers may recommend follow-up tests every 1-2 years to monitor progress and adjust treatment plans as necessary.

Is Exercise Safe for People with Osteoporosis?

Exercise can be safe and beneficial for individuals with osteoporosis, provided it is approached with caution. Low-impact, weight-bearing activities such as walking, dancing, and tai chi can improve bone strength while minimizing the risk of injury. It's important to consult with a healthcare provider or physical therapist to develop an exercise plan that considers individual capabilities and limitations, ensuring safety and effectiveness.

Incorporating strength training with light weights can also be advantageous, as it helps build muscle mass and enhances overall stability. Always listen to your body and make adjustments as needed, focusing on maintaining a consistent exercise routine that promotes bone health while prioritizing safety.

Conclusion

Summary of the Importance of Understanding Osteoporosis

Osteoporosis is a condition that weakens bones, making them fragile and more susceptible to fractures. Understanding osteoporosis is crucial as it affects millions of people worldwide, particularly older adults. By knowing how this condition develops, individuals can recognize its implications on bone health and take preventive measures early in life to maintain stronger bones. Awareness leads to informed decisions about lifestyle choices, nutrition, and exercise that can mitigate the risks associated with osteoporosis.

Recognizing the importance of bone health extends beyond just avoiding fractures; it contributes to overall well-being and independence as individuals age. Education about osteoporosis empowers people to understand the significance of maintaining bone density through proper nutrition, physical activity, and regular health check-ups. This knowledge serves as a foundation for fostering healthy habits that promote lifelong bone strength.

Encouragement to Take Proactive Steps for Bone Health

Taking proactive steps for bone health begins with incorporating a balanced diet rich in calcium and vitamin D. Foods such as dairy products, leafy greens, nuts, and fatty fish are excellent sources of these nutrients. Additionally, consider fortified foods and supplements if dietary intake is insufficient. Establishing healthy eating habits in early adulthood sets the stage for optimal bone density and strength as one ages.

Engaging in regular weight-bearing exercises, such as walking, jogging, or strength training, is vital for stimulating bone growth and maintenance. Aim for at least 30 minutes of exercise most days of the week, incorporating activities that strengthen muscles and improve balance.

Importance of Seeking Professional Guidance and Support

Consulting healthcare professionals is essential for individuals concerned about osteoporosis. Physicians, dietitians, and physical therapists can provide personalized assessments, recommendations, and support tailored to individual needs. Regular check-ups allow for early detection of bone density issues, enabling timely intervention and management strategies that can significantly impact health outcomes.

Additionally, support groups and educational programs can offer valuable resources and encouragement. These platforms connect individuals with similar concerns, fostering a community where experiences and strategies for managing osteoporosis are shared. Seeking guidance from professionals and peer support can empower individuals to take charge of their bone health, leading to a more informed and proactive approach to prevention and management.